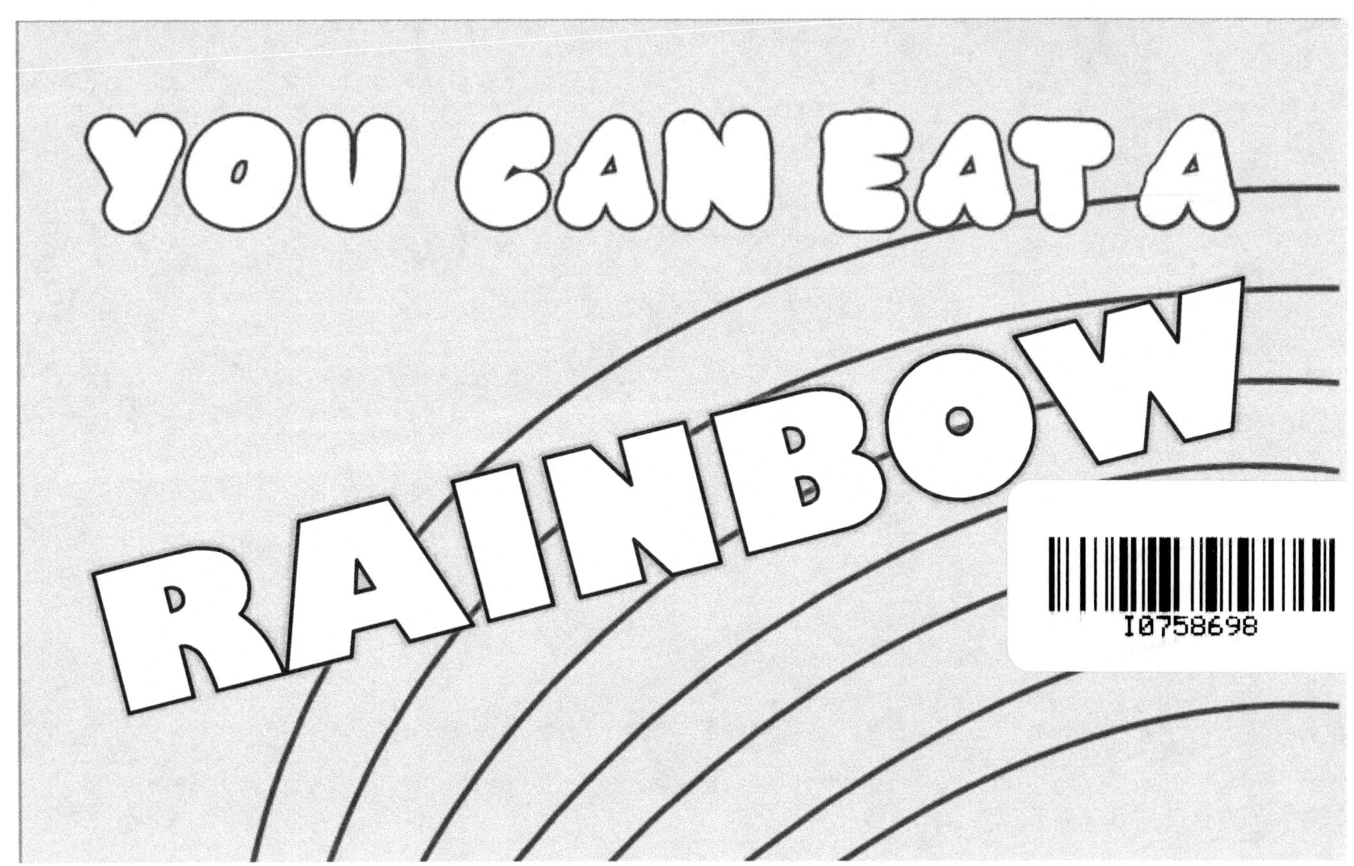

Written by Kim Turinske

Illustrated by Kristi Atwater

Graphic Support by Gabbie Hirsch

This is a coloring book written by a family practice doctor who specializes in weight loss. This book makes eating fun for kids and teaches them to eat a variety of fruits and vegetables while coloring. It also explains why it is important to eat fruits and vegetables. It's a great book to teach kids about healthy eating. It's a win for parents and kids.

2023 All Rights Reserved ISBN 9798854100205

You probably think eating a rainbow, can't be done,
but I am here to tell you it can be fun!
There are rainbows of colors
in your grocery store,
look carefully and
you find many more.

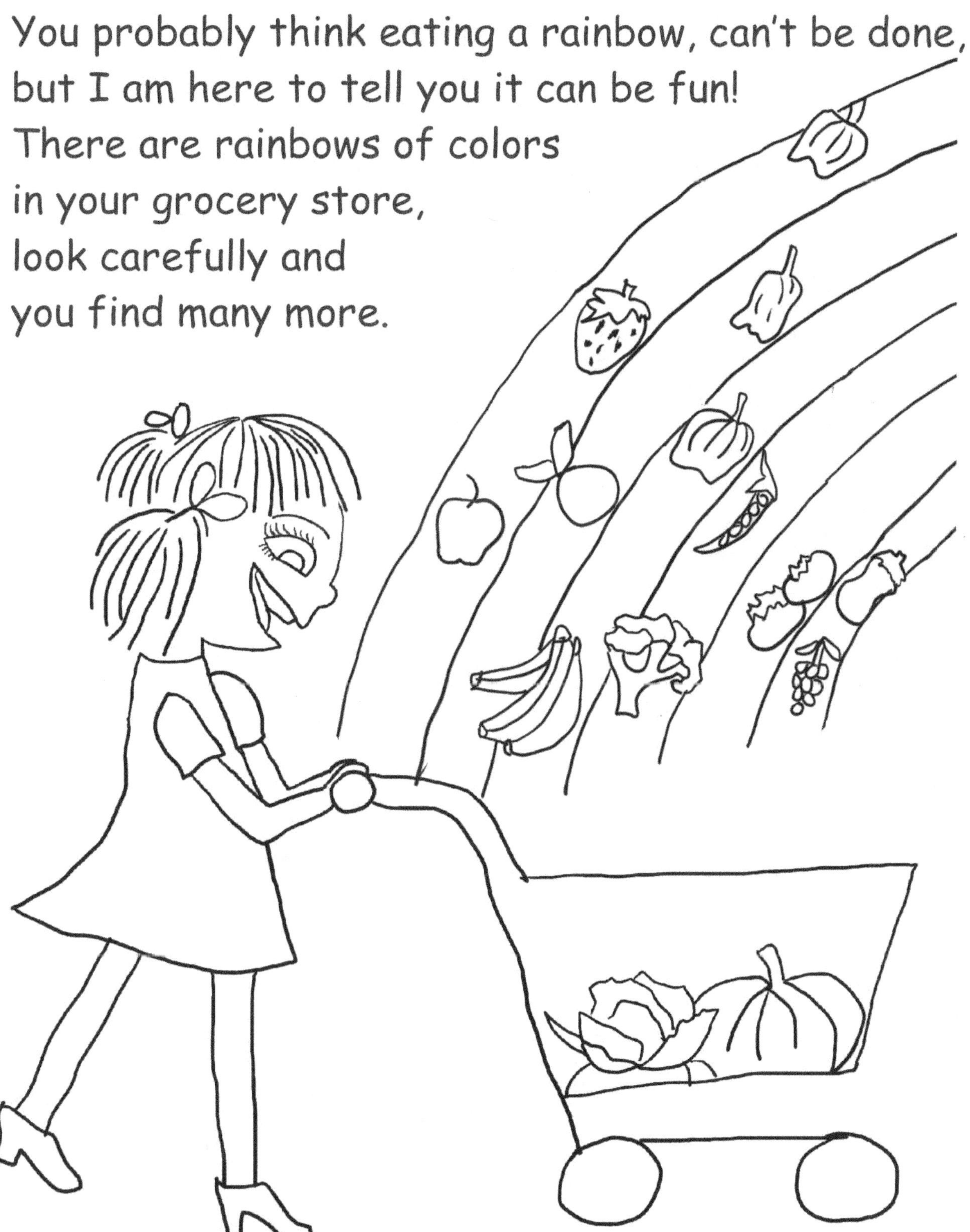

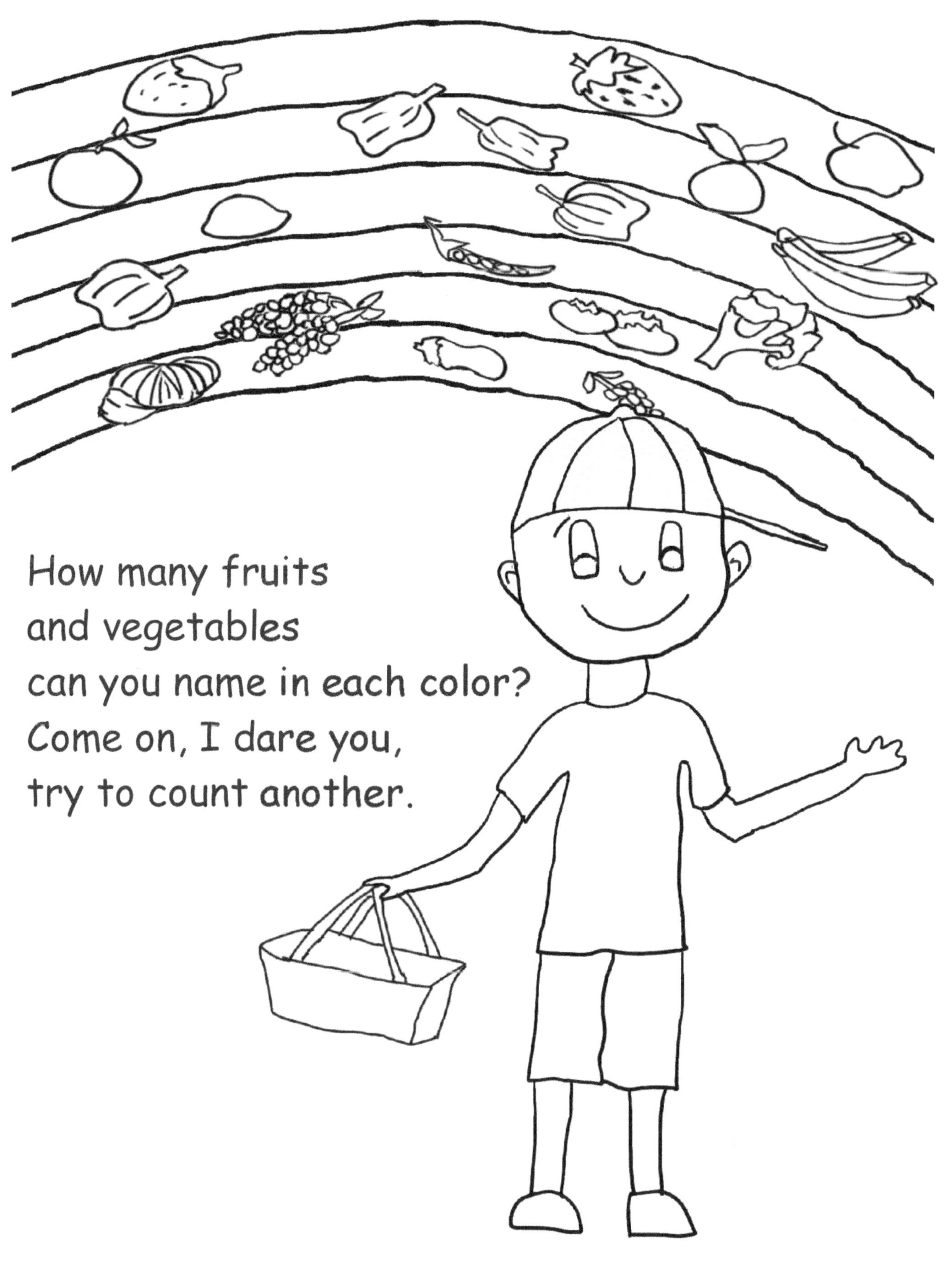
How many fruits
and vegetables
can you name in each color?
Come on, I dare you,
try to count another.

Here we go, get it in your head,
you can eat a rainbow,
and the first color is
RED!

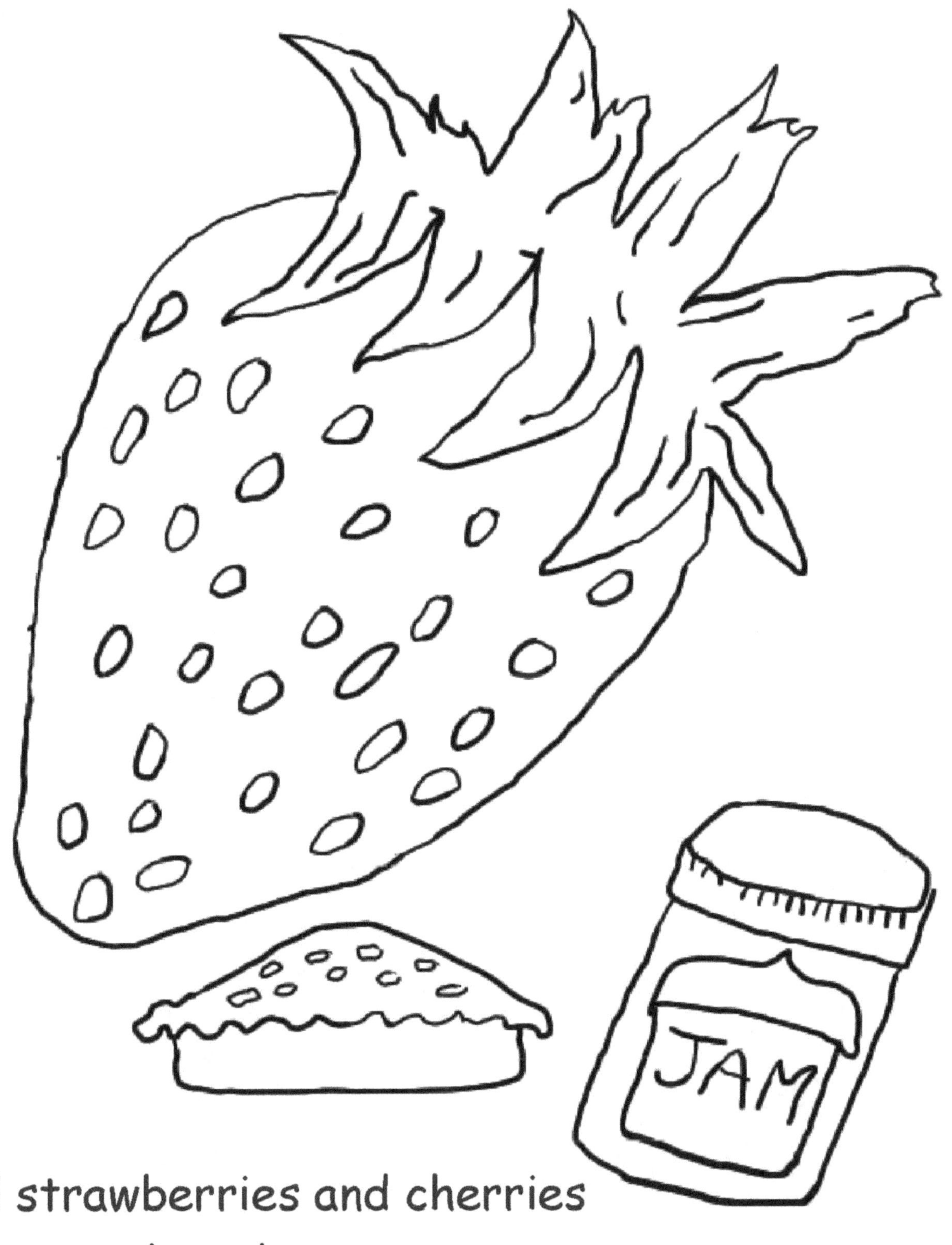

Red strawberries and cherries
are super to eat.
Have them fresh, or in yogurt,
but dipped in dark chocolate,they can't be beat.

Tomatoes are tart, but they help your heart!

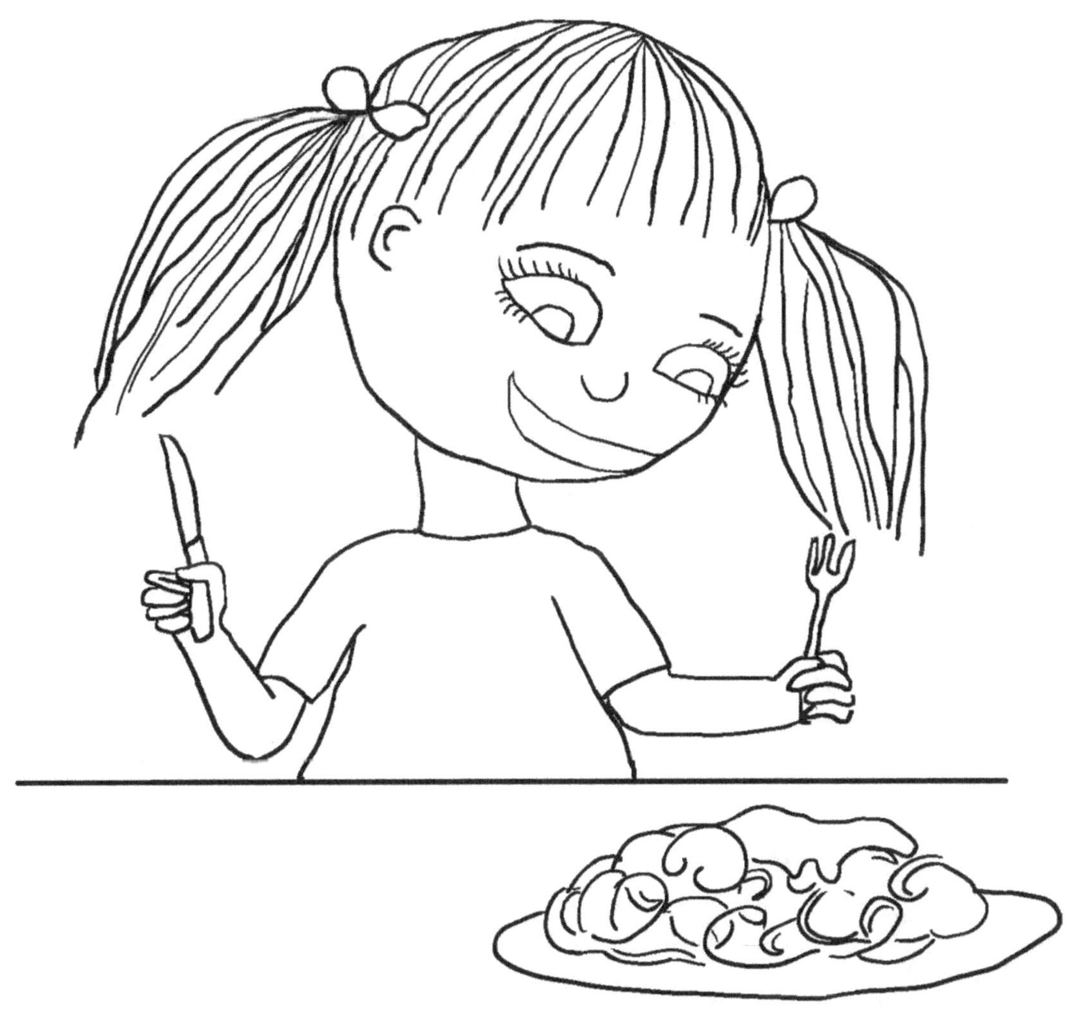

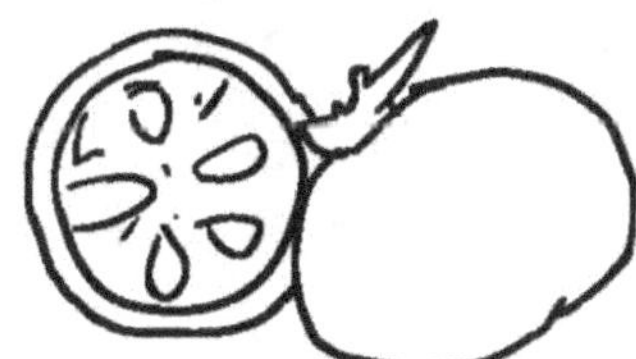

Eat them in Spaghetti!

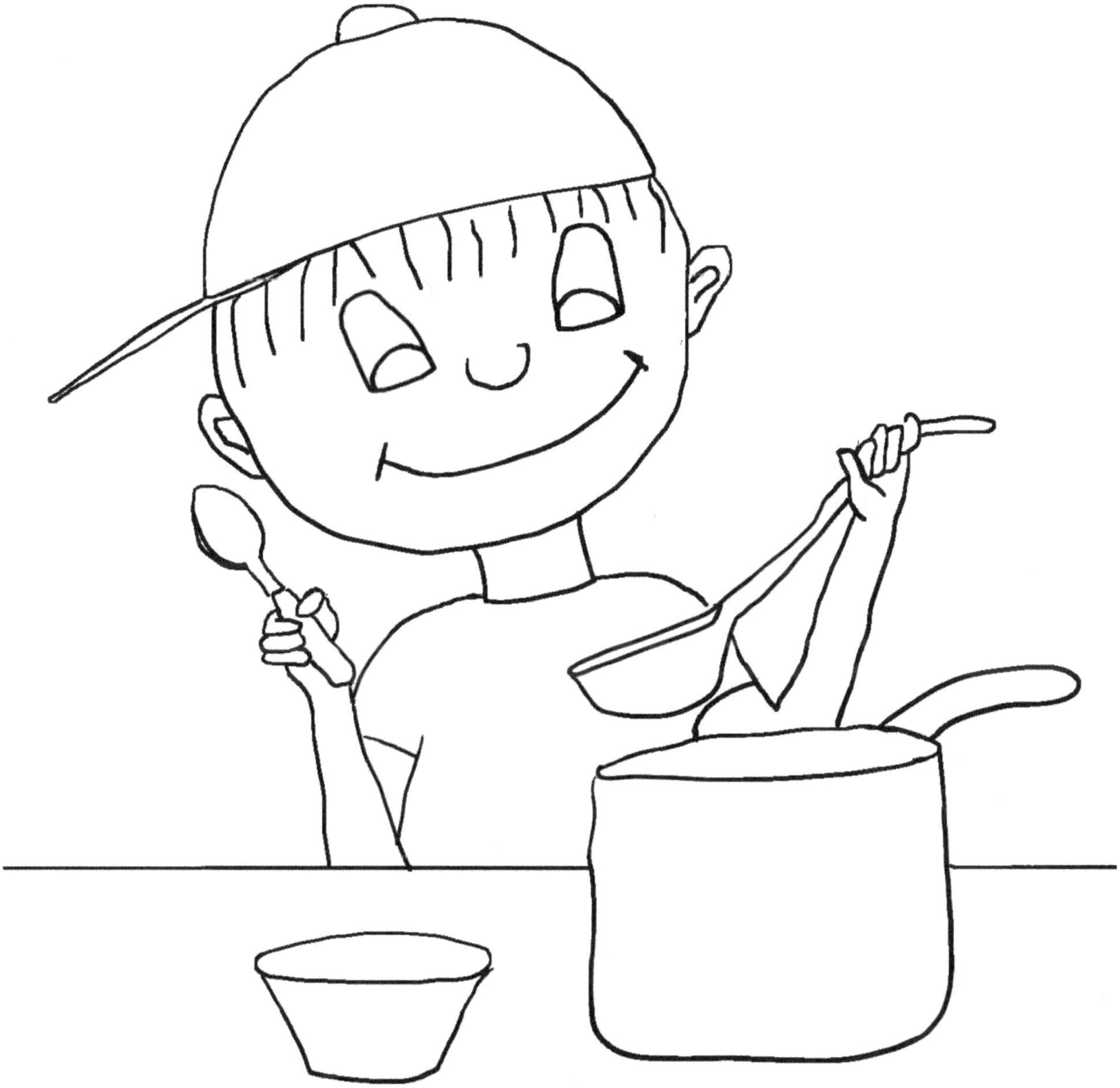

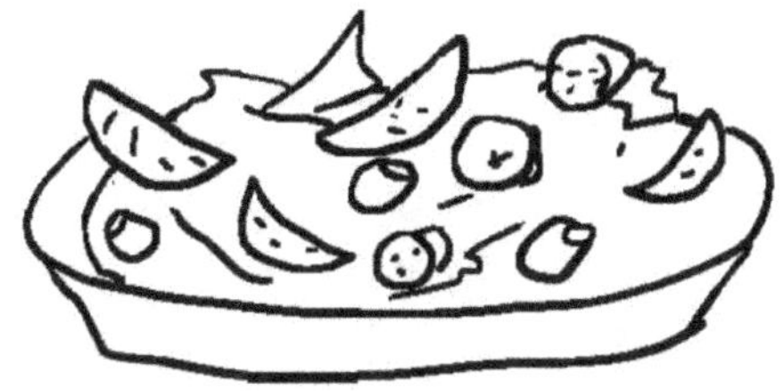

Or, have them in soup,
  they are great on tacos,
    so take a big scoop!

The next color of the rainbow
for you to try is
YELLOW.

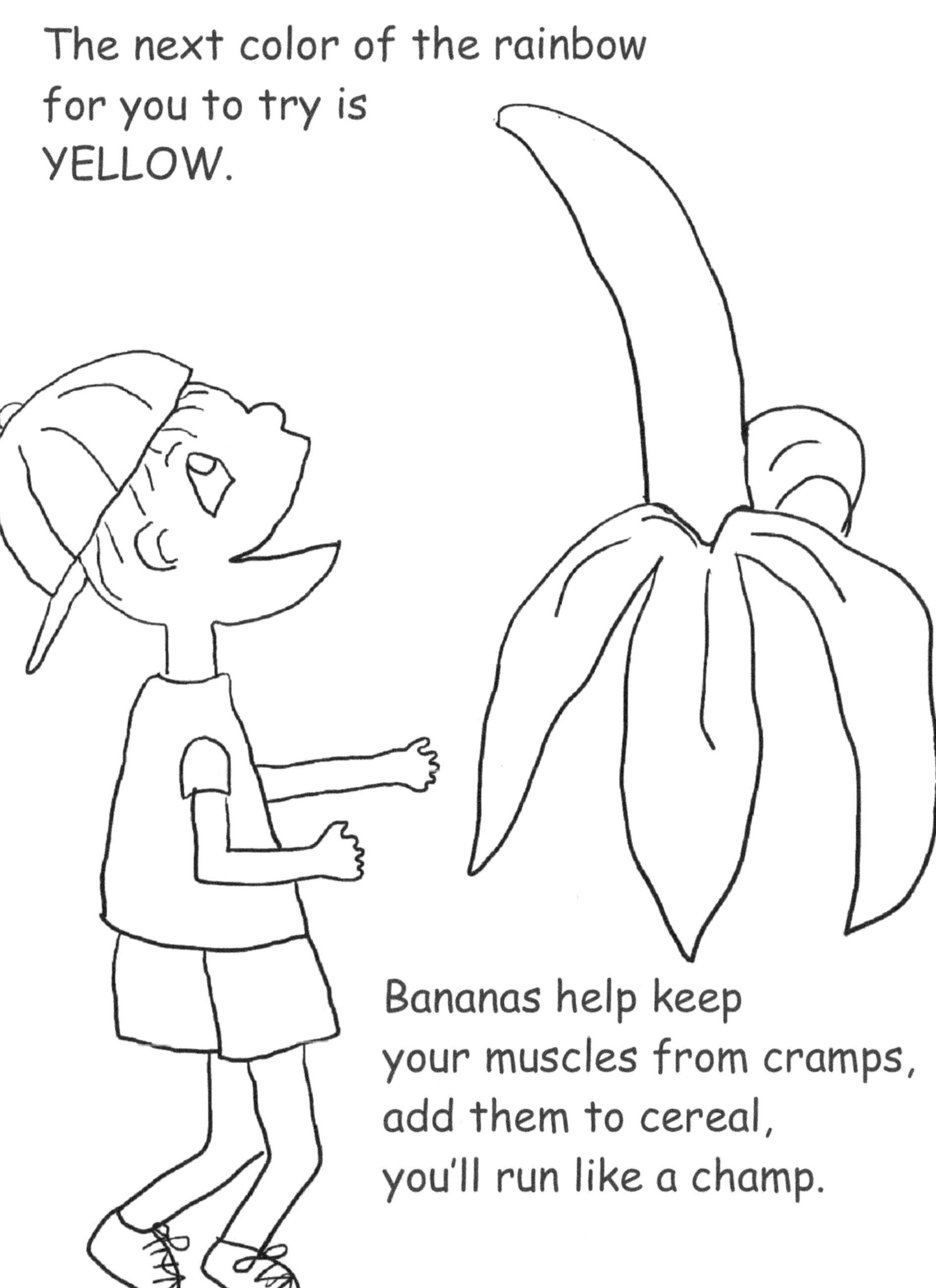

Bananas help keep
your muscles from cramps,
add them to cereal,
you'll run like a champ.

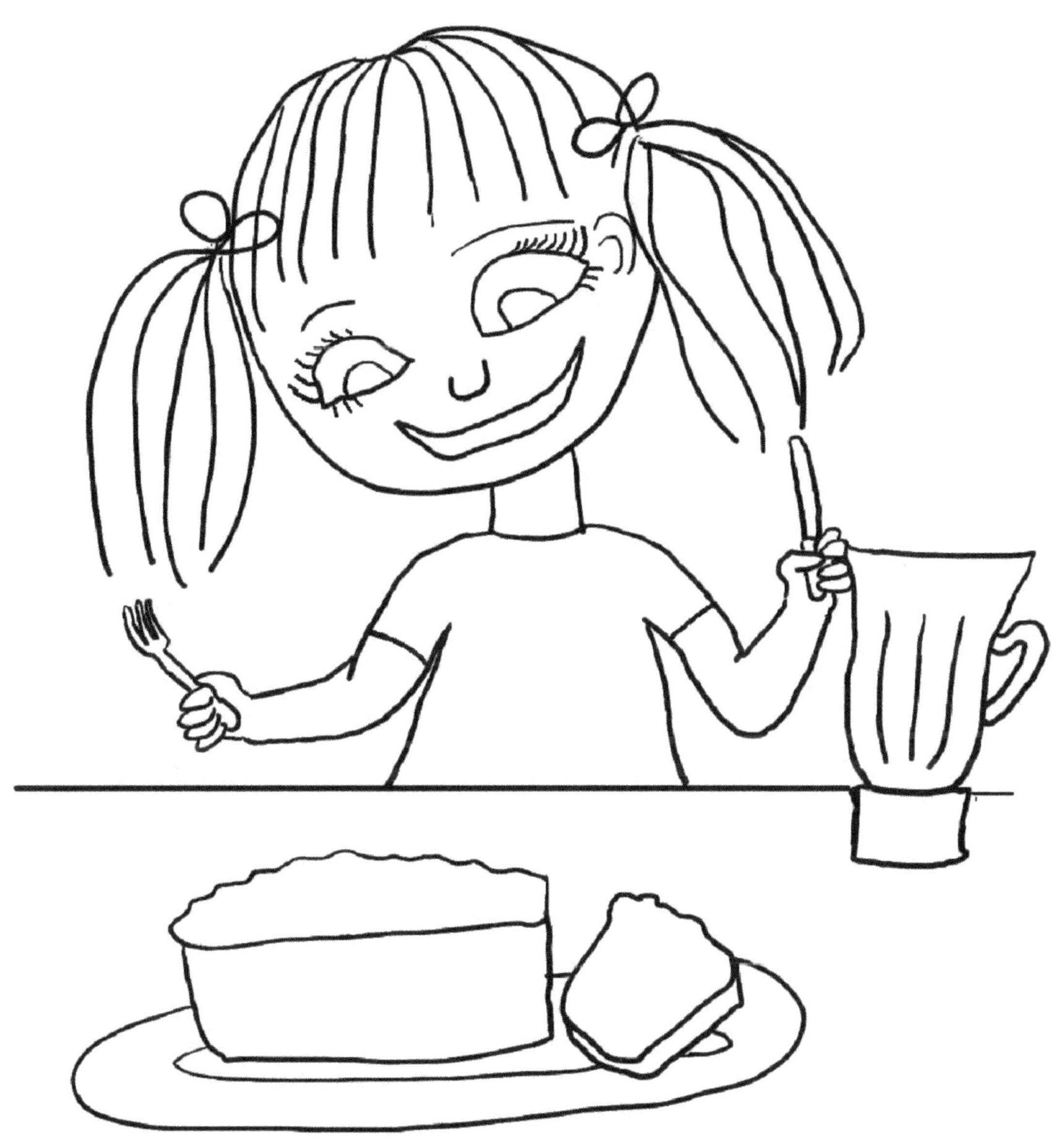

You can put them in shakes,
or bake them in bread,
or have after school
for a snack, instead.

Pineapple is incredibly sweet,
fresh from Hawaii,
it's the ultimate treat!

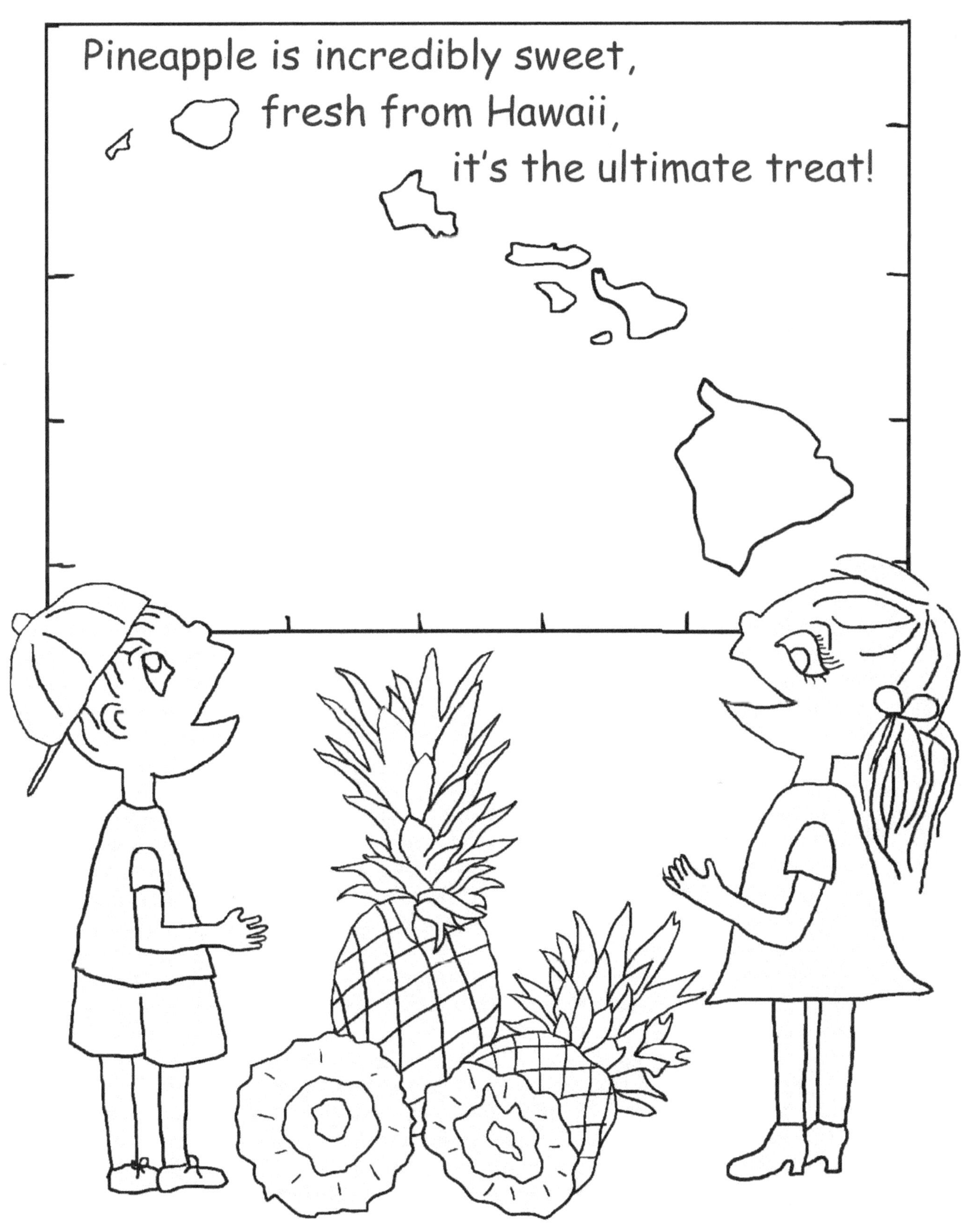

What is another color in a rainbow?
Oh, that's right, it is PINK!

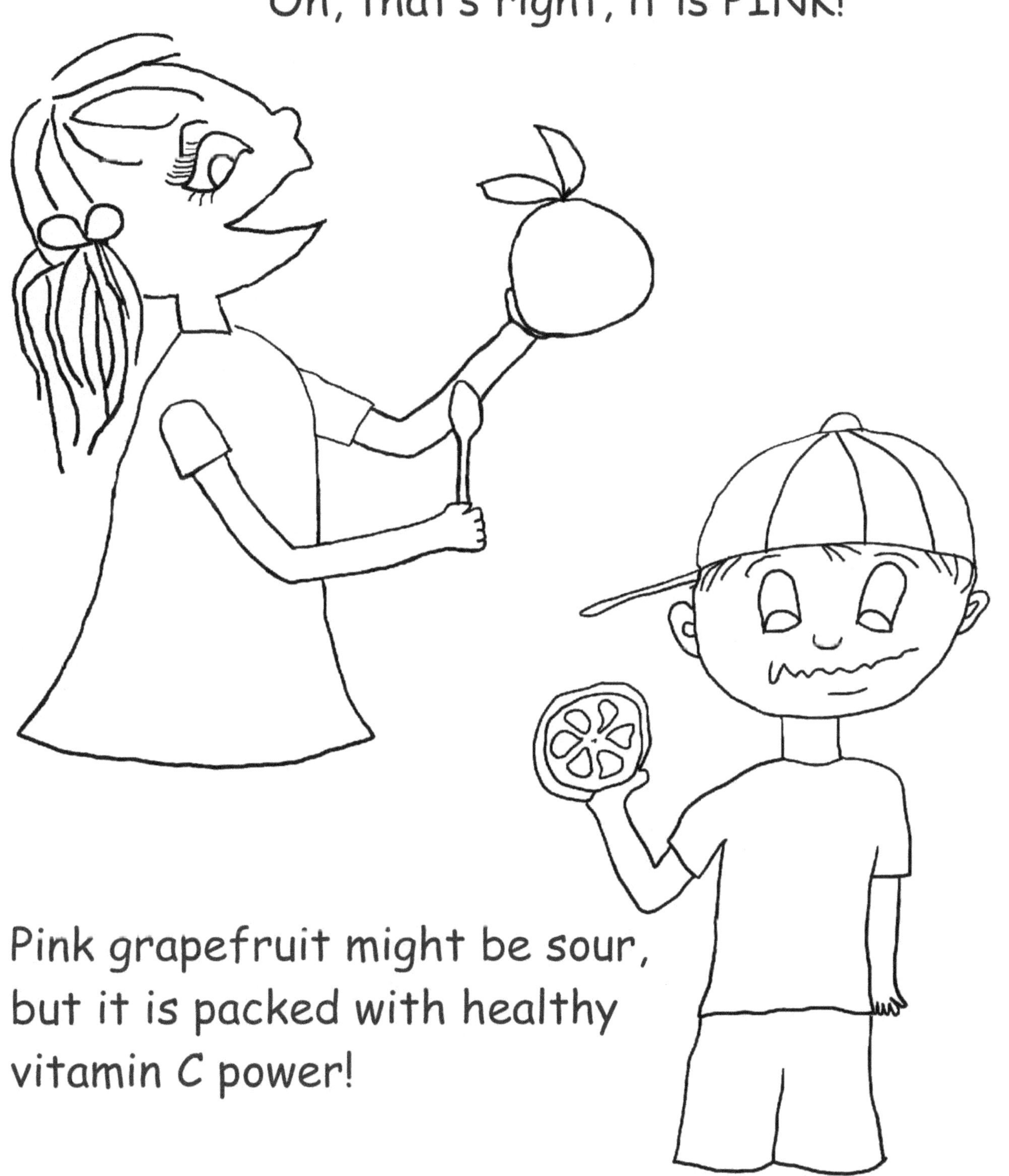

Pink grapefruit might be sour,
but it is packed with healthy
vitamin C power!

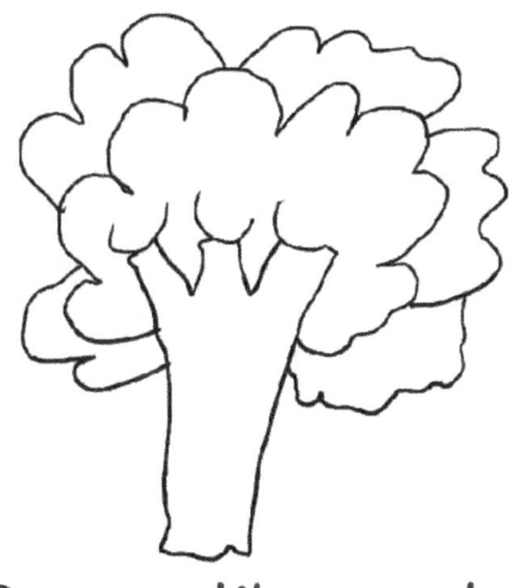

I know I'm forgetting a color.
What could it be?
That's right, it's GREEN!

Broccoli's good at keeping cancer away,
so eat some every day.
Eat it raw, or with dip,

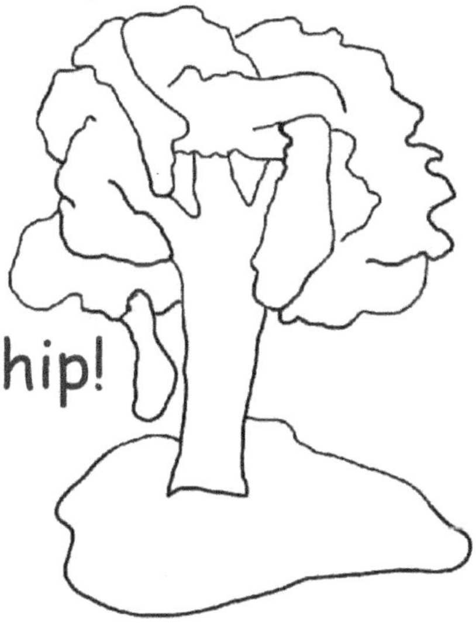

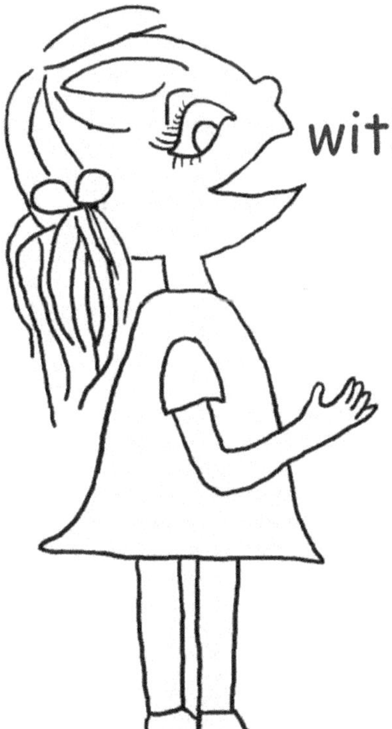

with cheese sauce, it is hip!

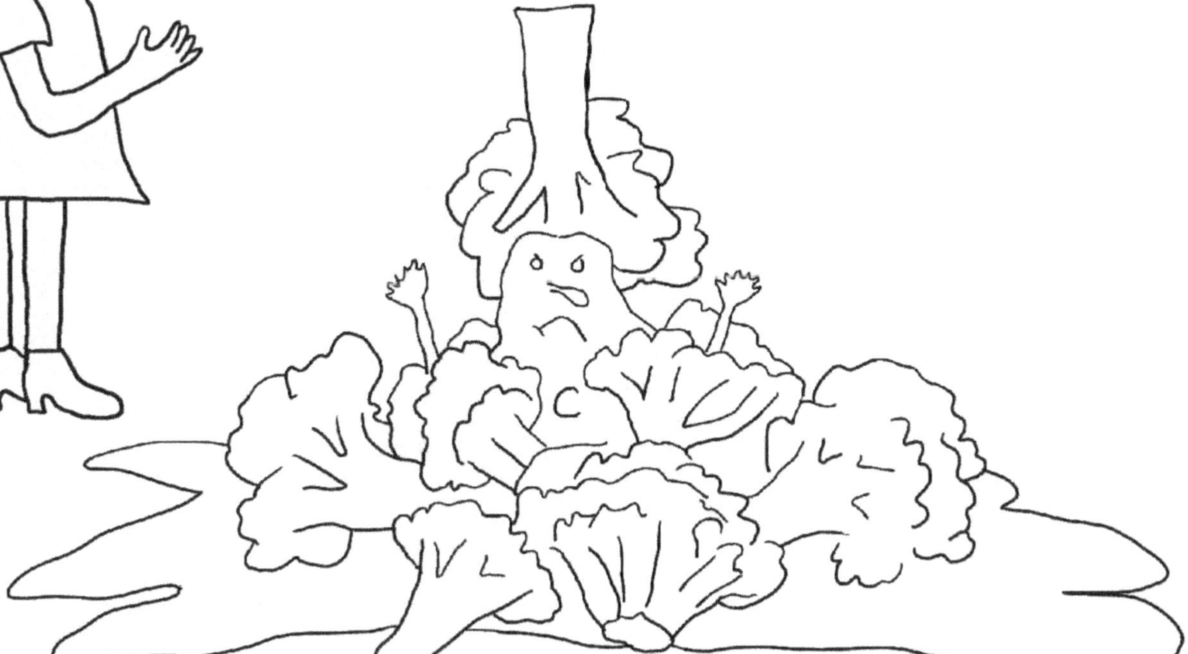

Leafy greens like spinach and lettuce have vitamin K, which helps keep cuts from bleeding away.

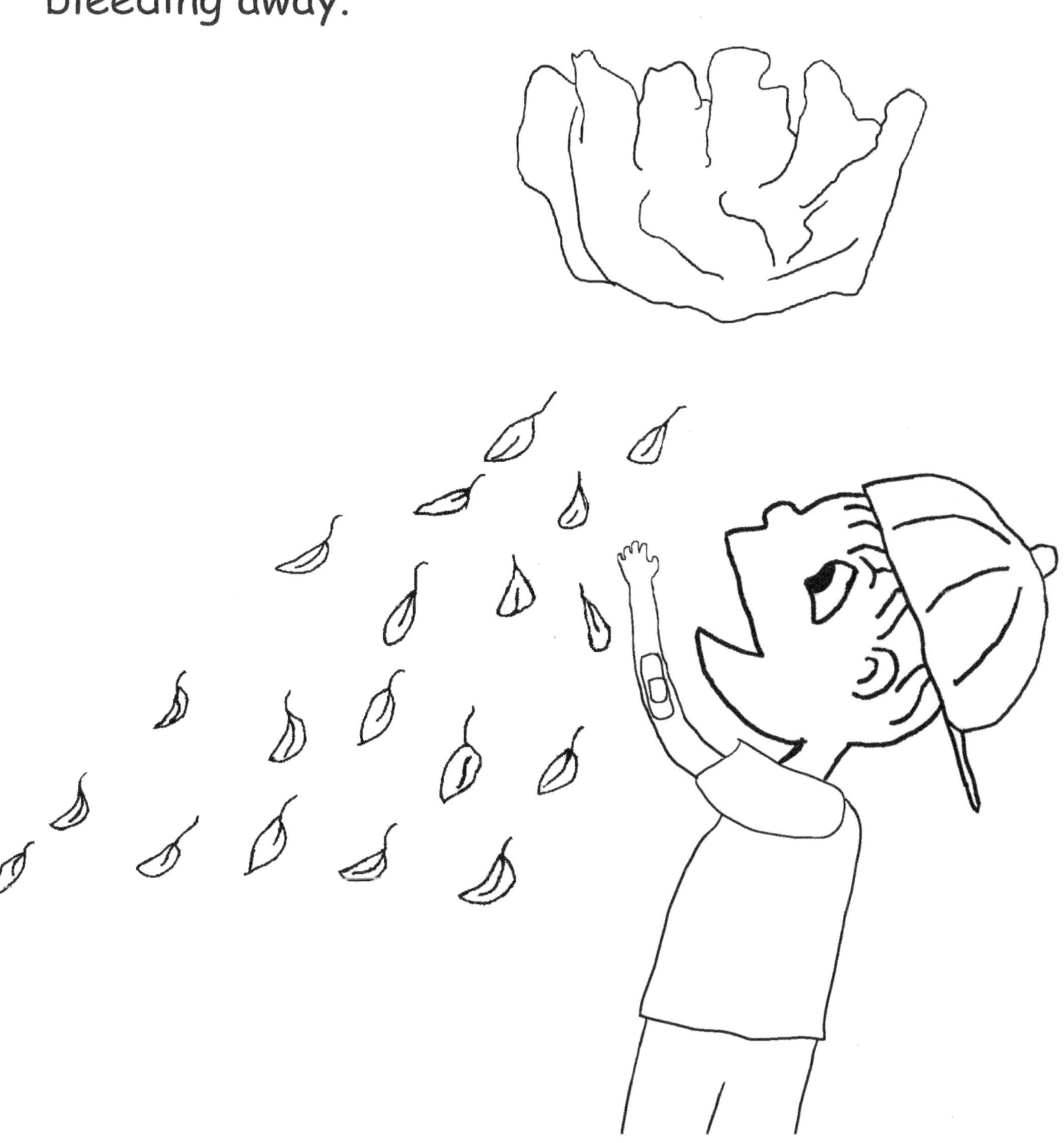

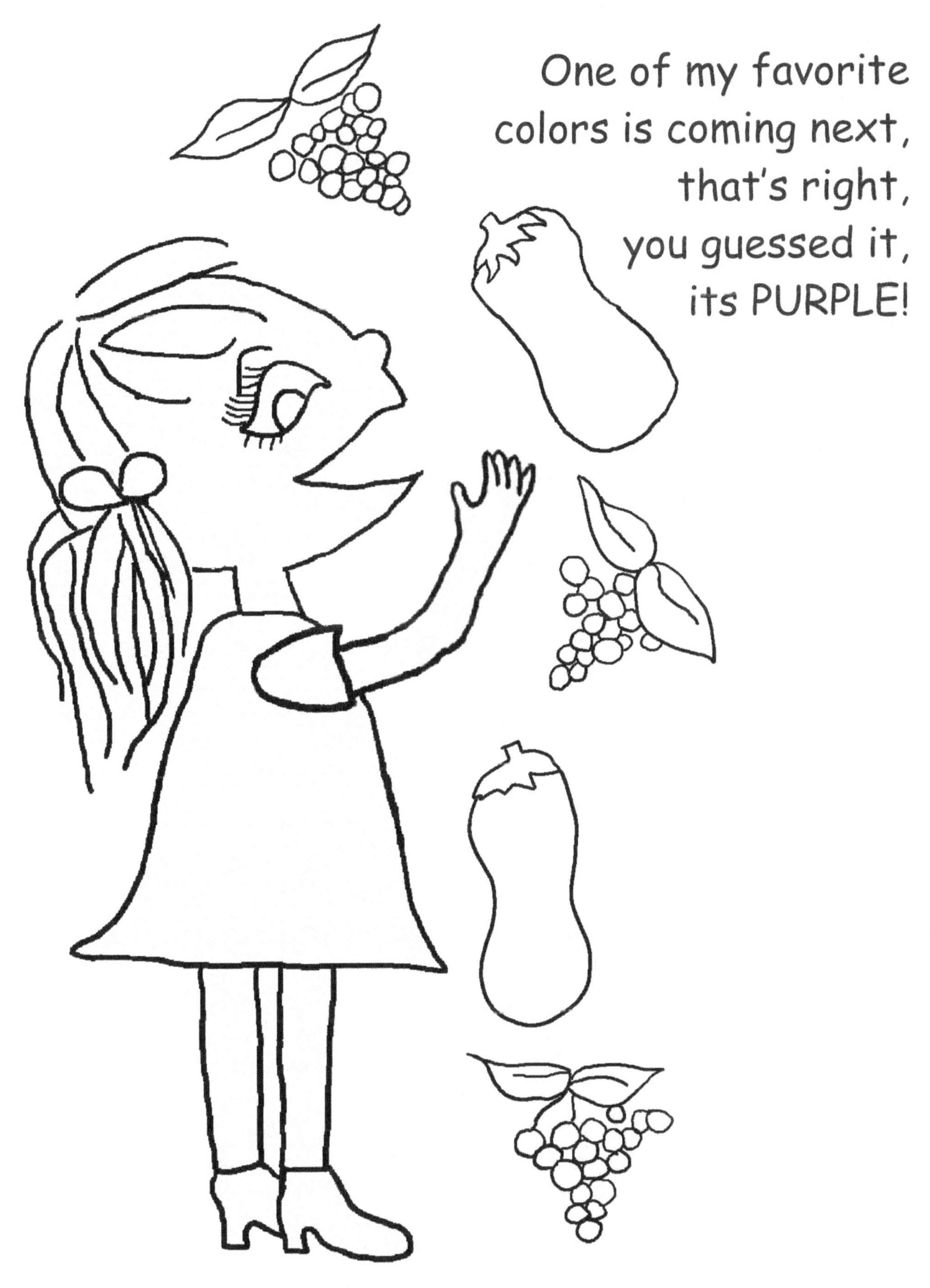

One of my favorite
colors is coming next,
that's right,
you guessed it,
its PURPLE!

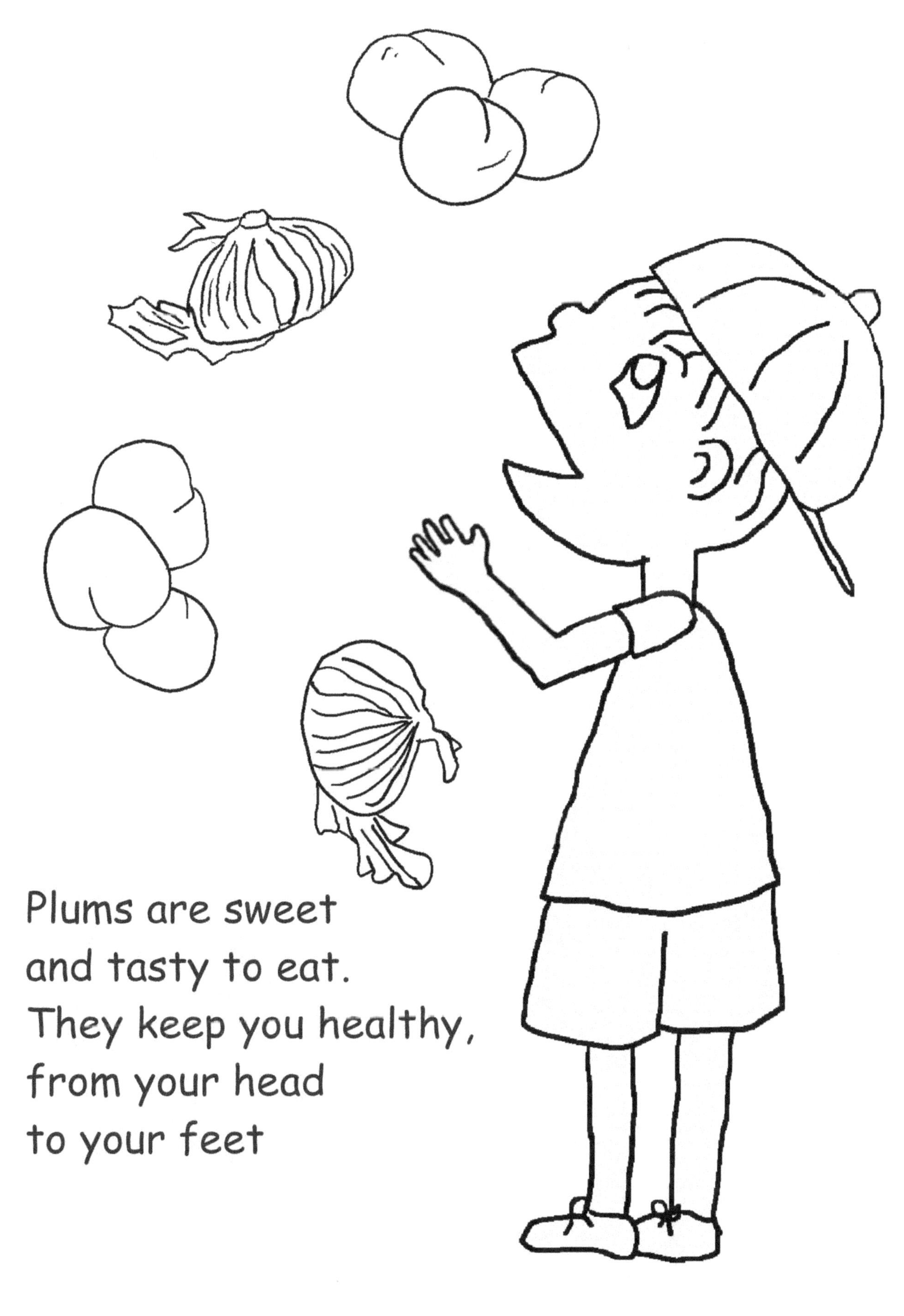

Plums are sweet
and tasty to eat.
They keep you healthy,
from your head
to your feet

There is one more color, ORANGE you glad?
It will keep you from being sick, which is bad.

Oranges help keep you from getting ill,
they are good in juice
with a little ice for chill.

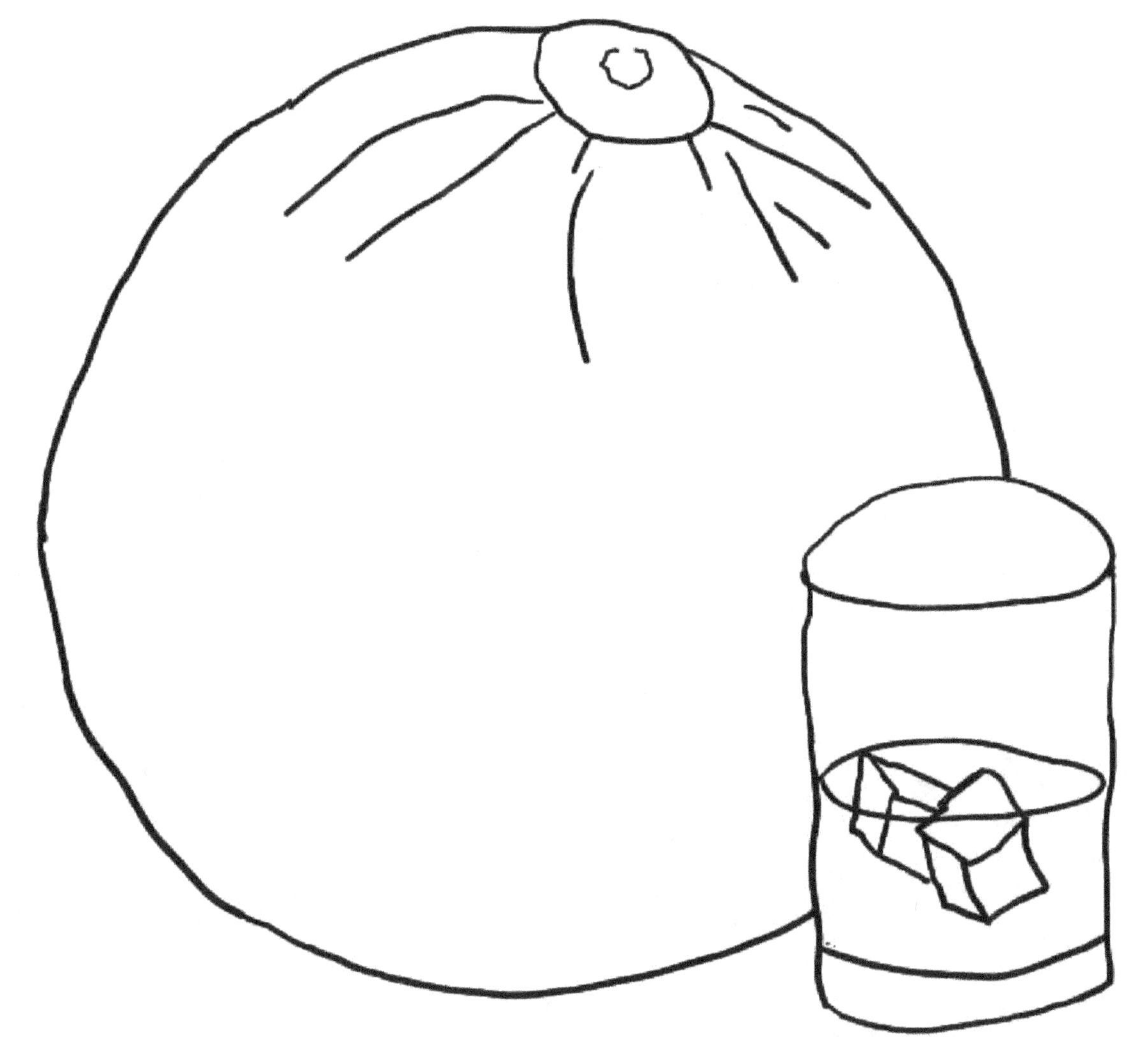

"Try me, Mr. Mango, I'm so good,
I'll make you Tango!"

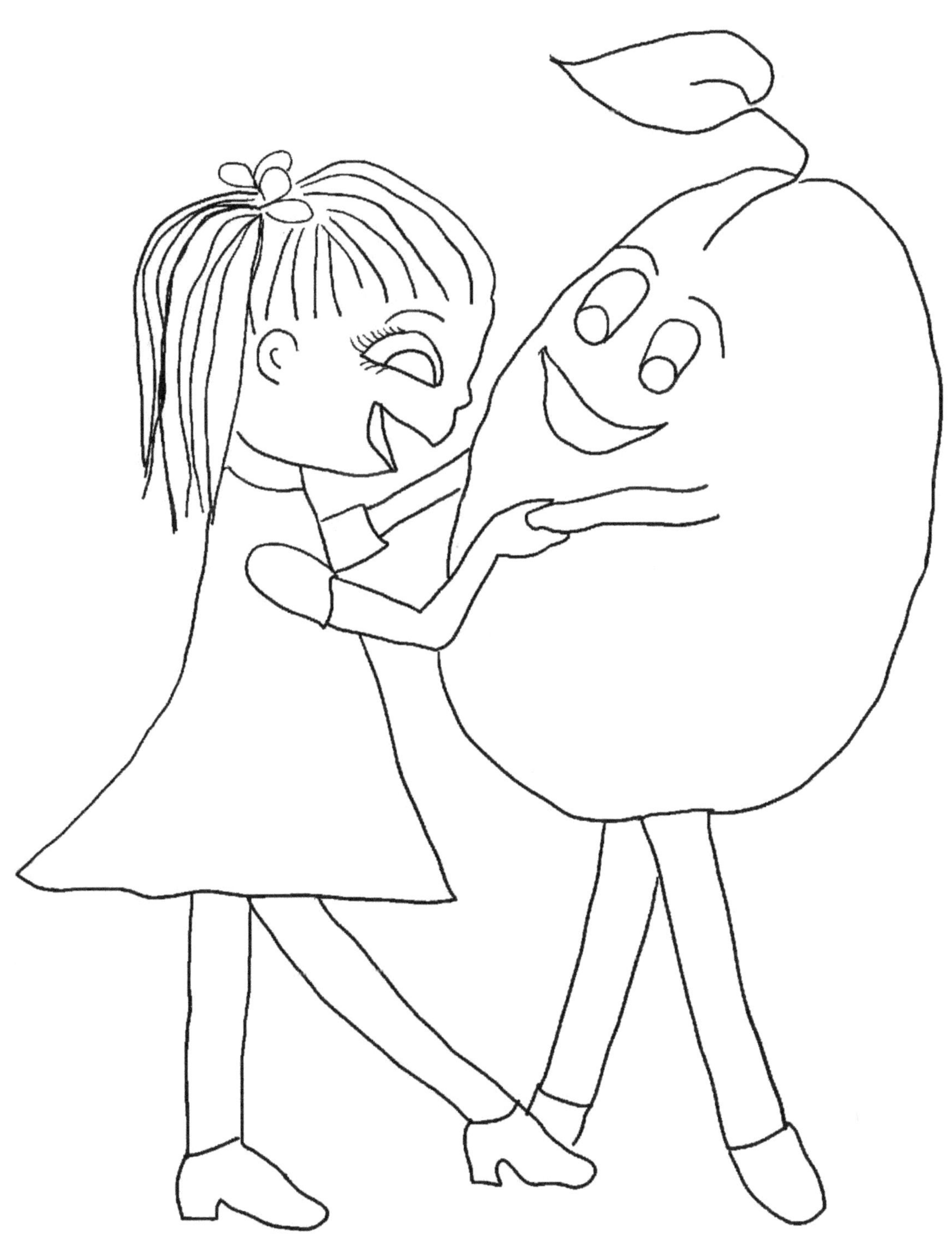

I'm a carrot, please pick me up,
I help you to see!
Carrots help you see at night,
and in old age help you
keep your sight.

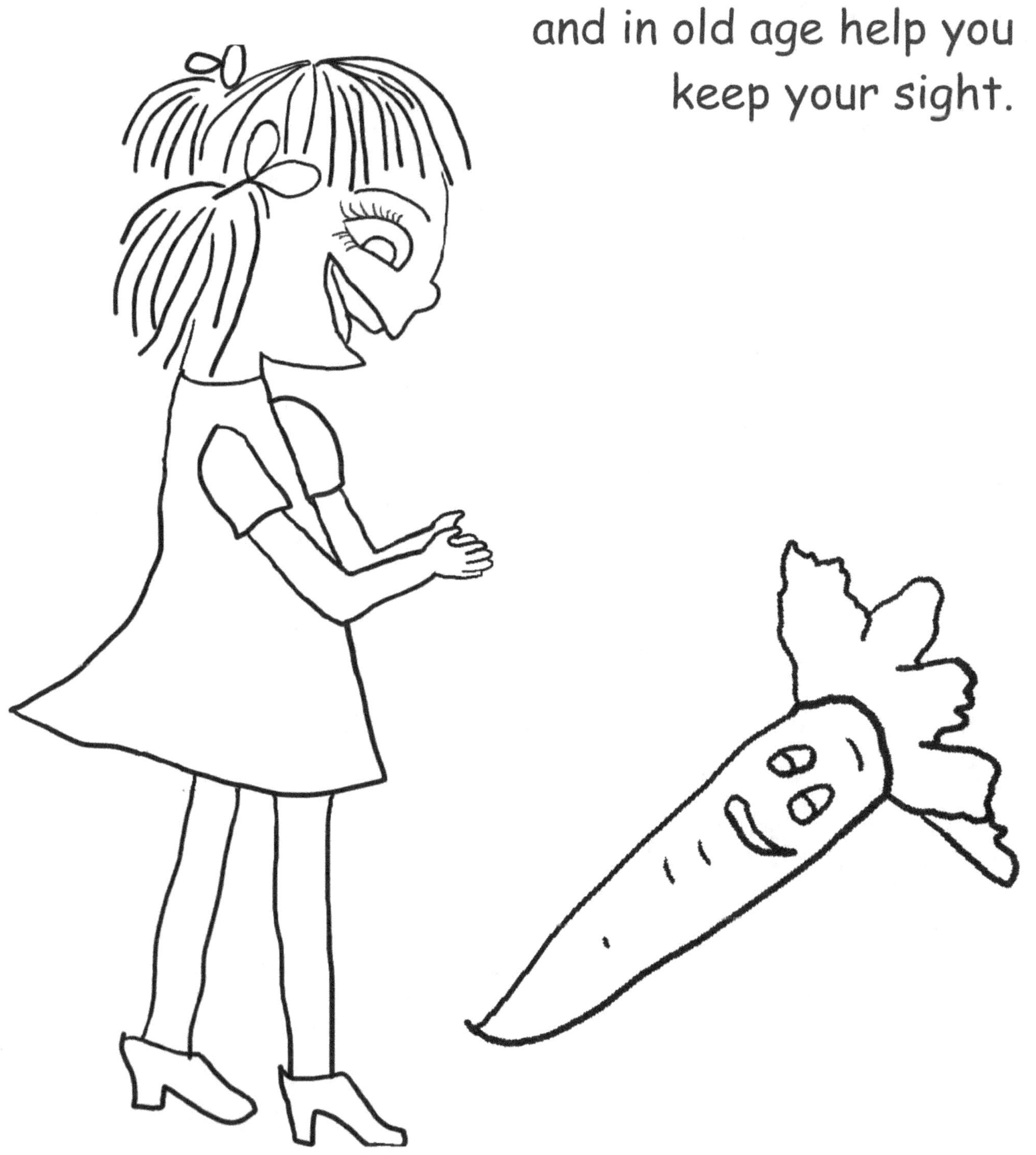

Put them in cake, or have them with dip,
or add them to soup and take a sip.

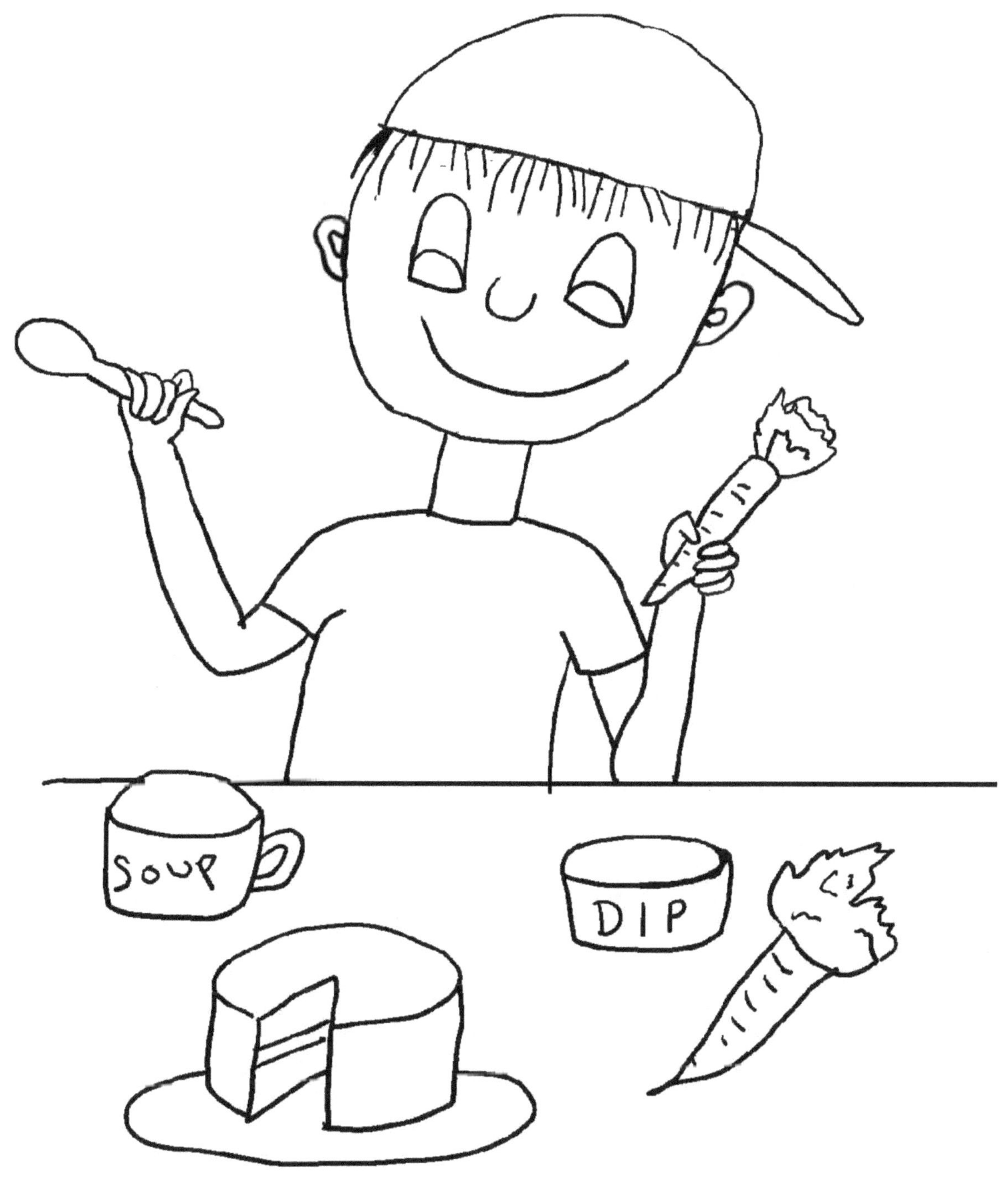

My neighbors the squash and pumpkins
are sweet, baked with brown sugar they can't
be beat.

Here is some advice for

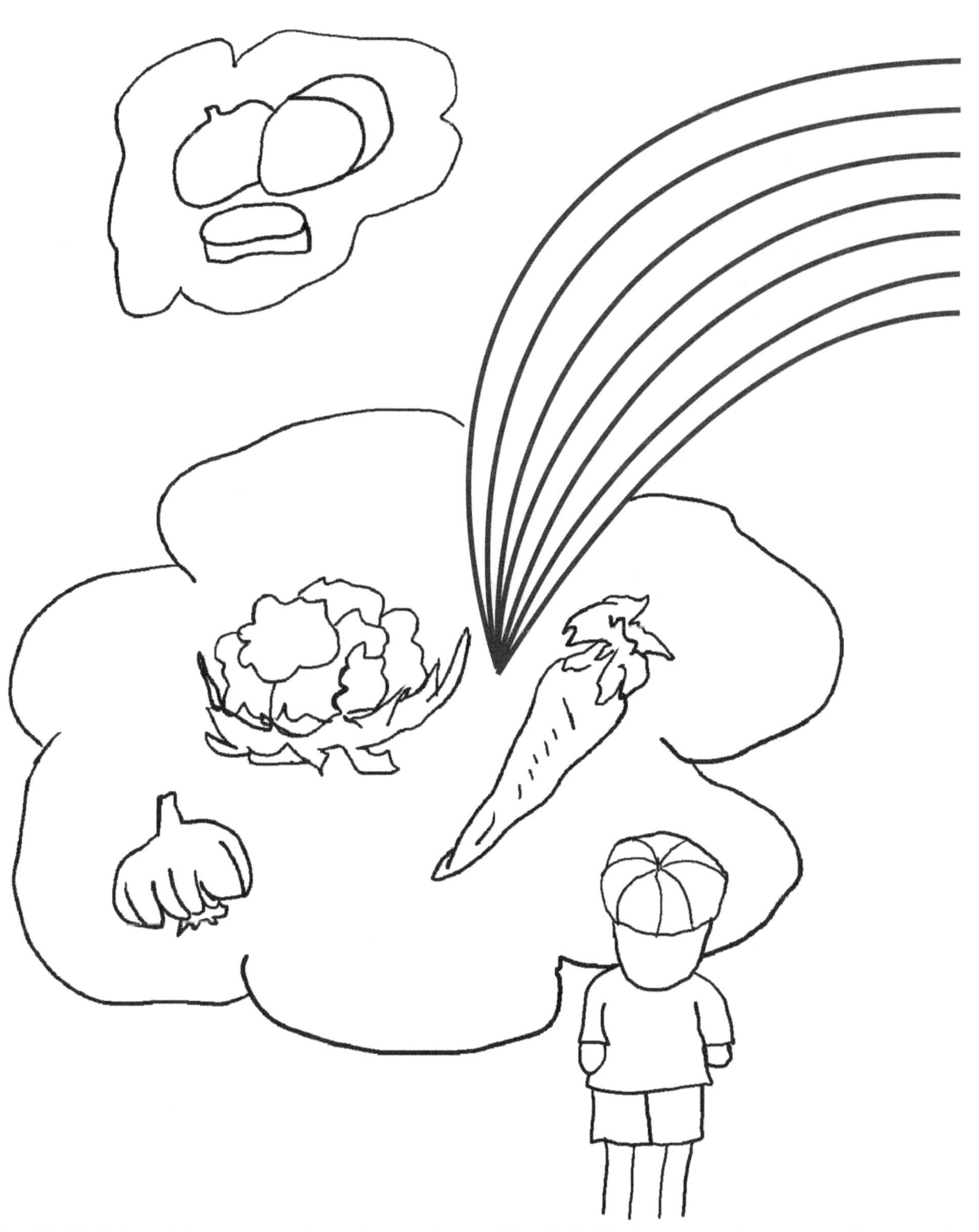

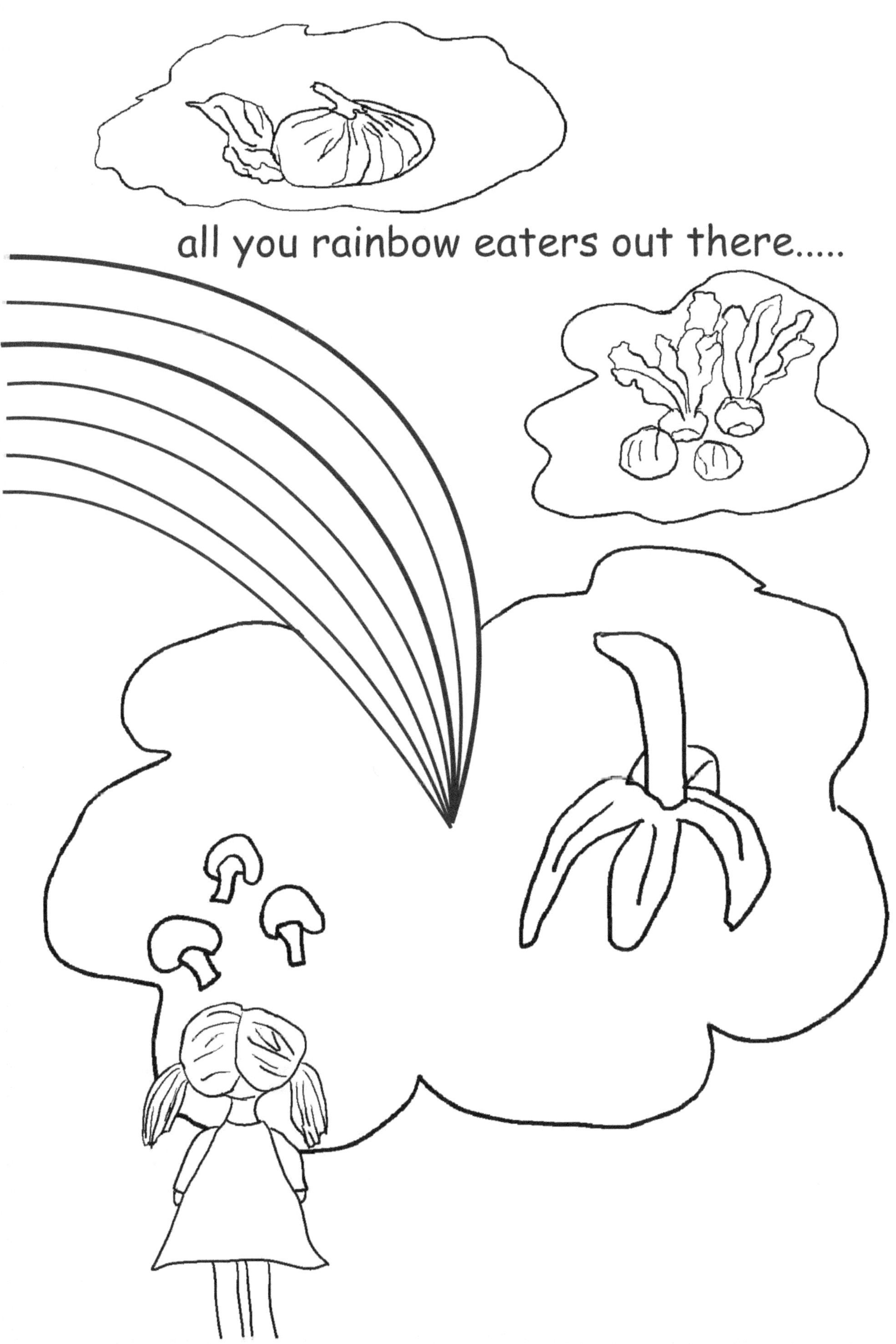
all you rainbow eaters out there.....

Each time you eat, ask yourself,
 "what does this food do?" If there is
no good answer, put it down say " Ka-Poo!"
Candy bars, cookies, french fries and pop,
pizza and chips, please don't put them
too often to your lips.

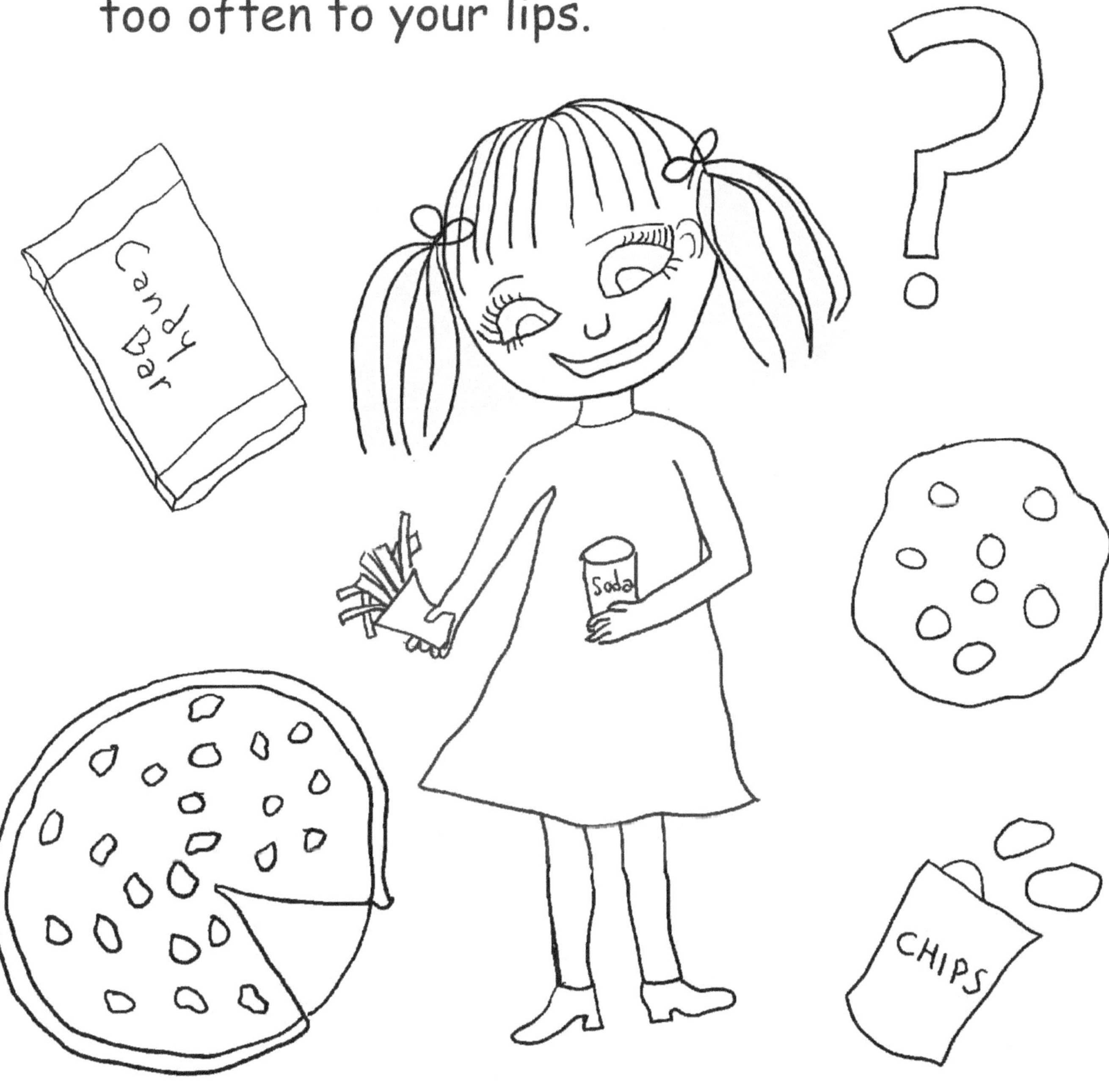

Don't eat fried foods like fries,
they plug up your heart, "'cuz for that,
there is no replacement part!"
 Your body uses food as fuel to make it run.
With unhealthy food it will break down,
which is no fun.

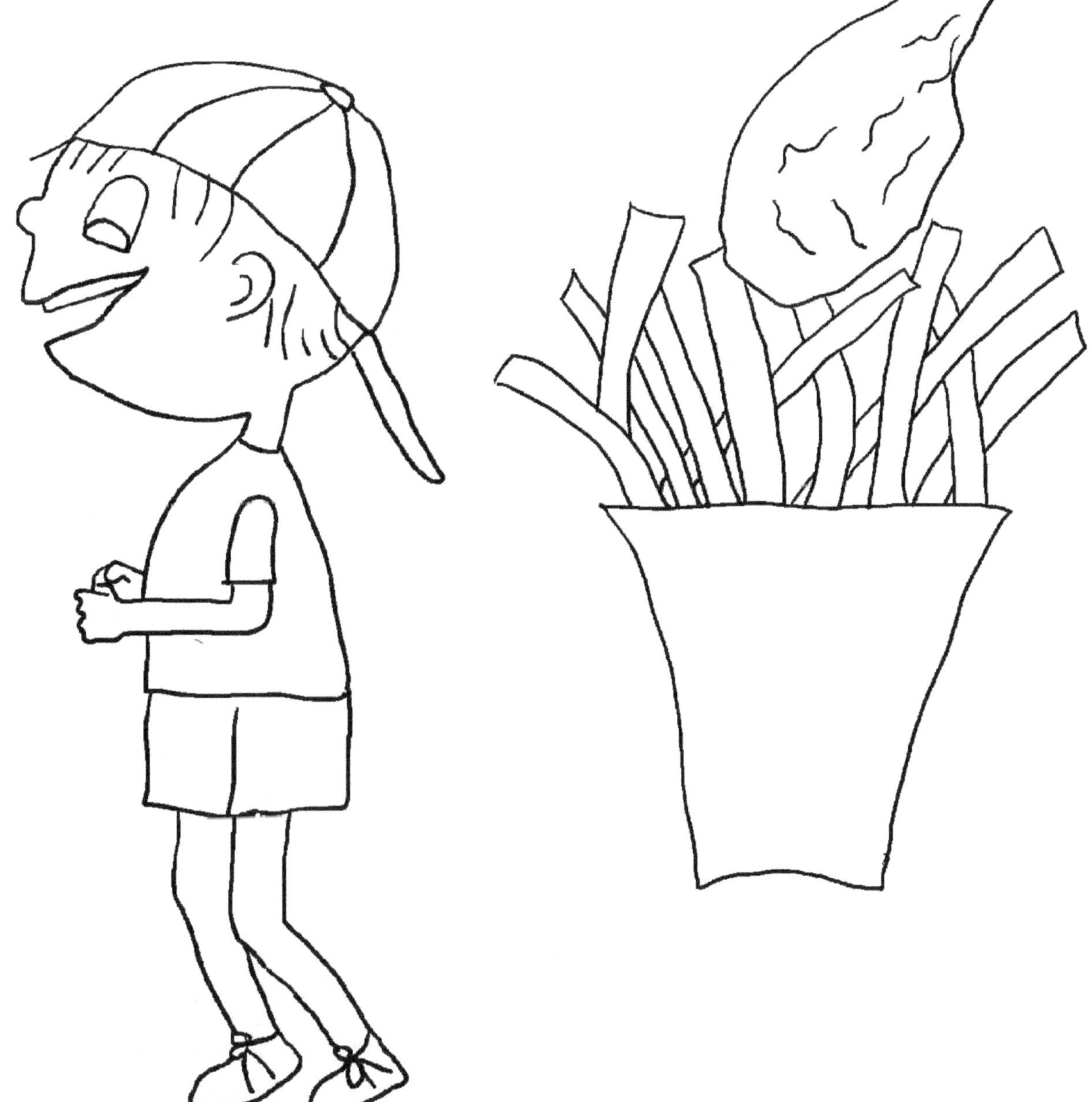

Every Color of the rainbow
in fruits and vegetables
has a different job to do.
Some help you see,
some help you pooh.

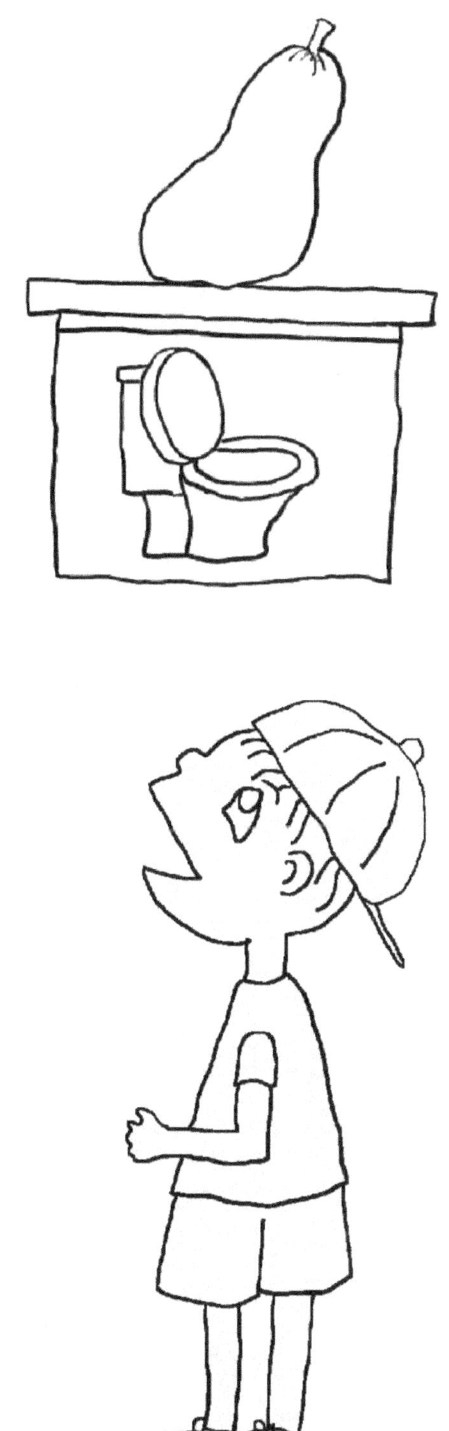

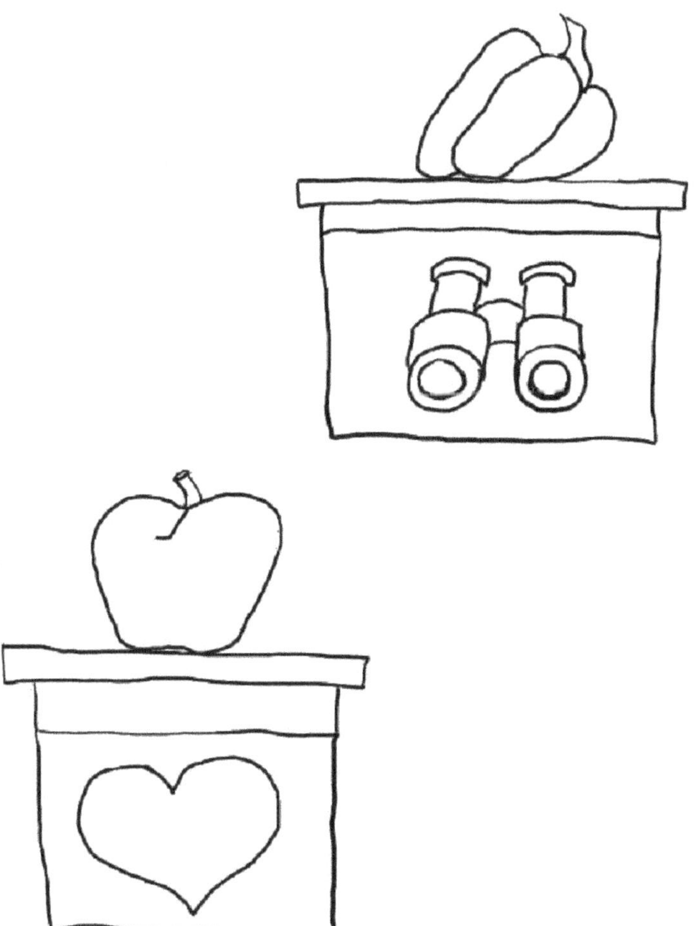

Some keep sickness at bay,
some keep cancer away.
Some keep your heart strong,
some help you sing a song!

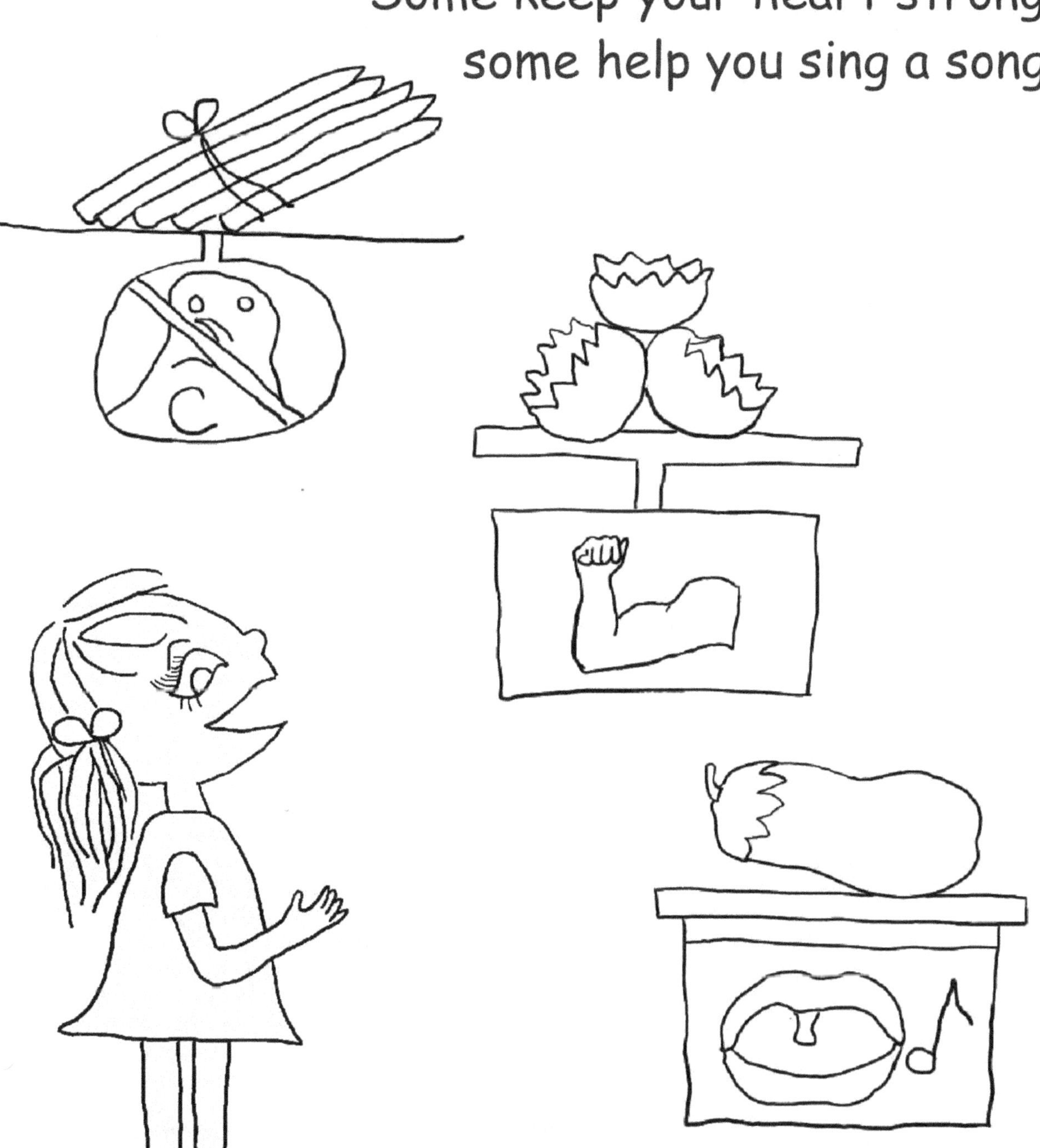

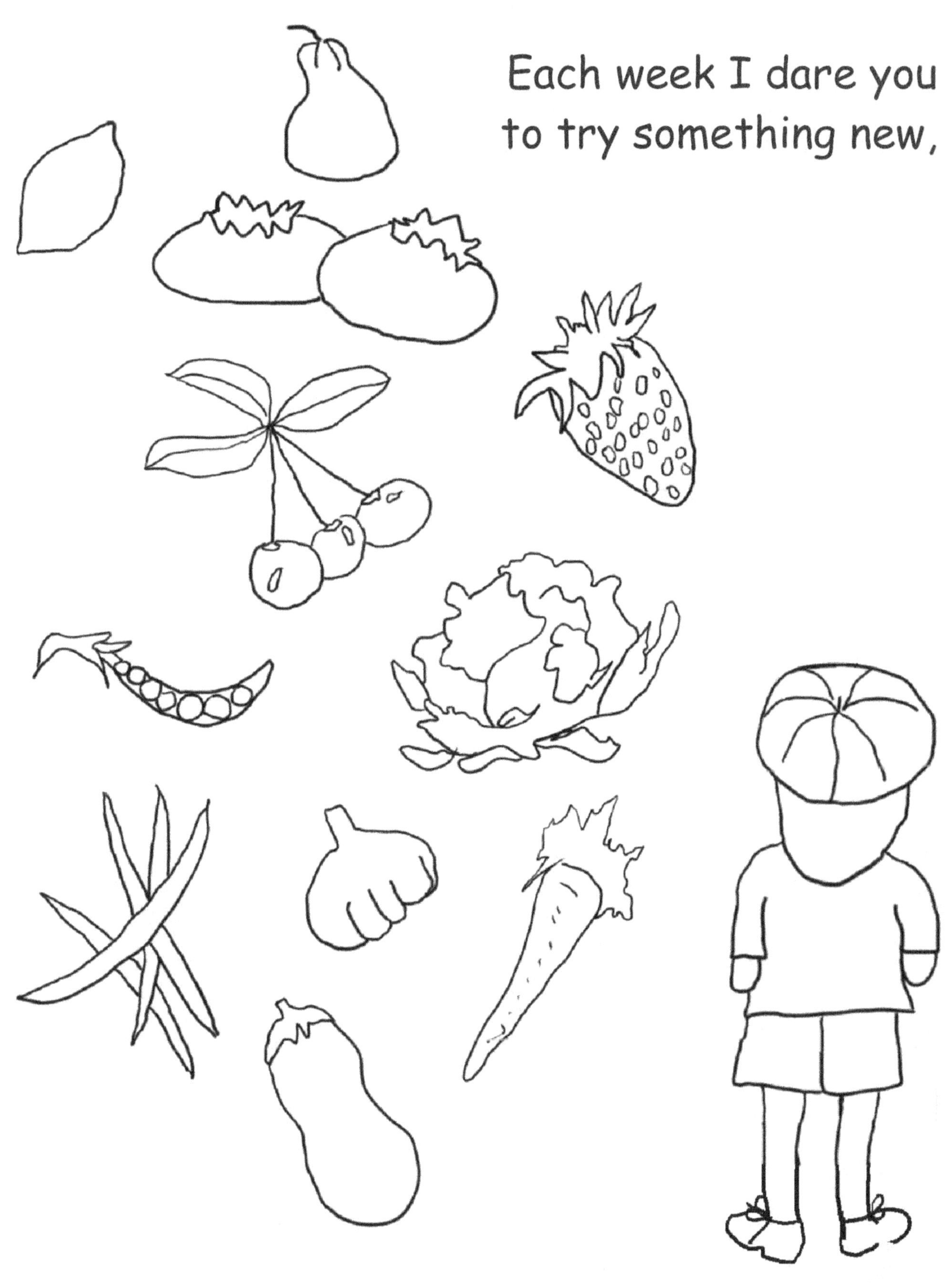

Each week I dare you
to try something new,

you'll feel good, stay healthy,
and be the best you!

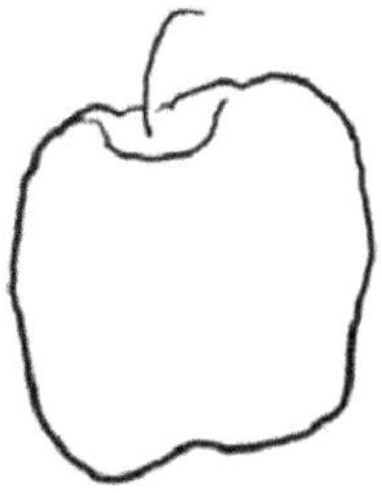

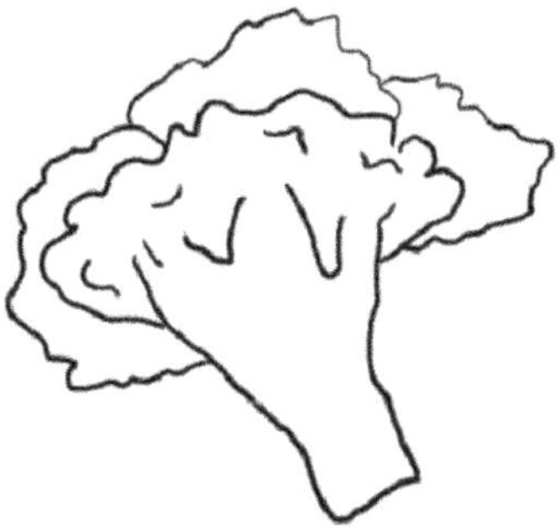

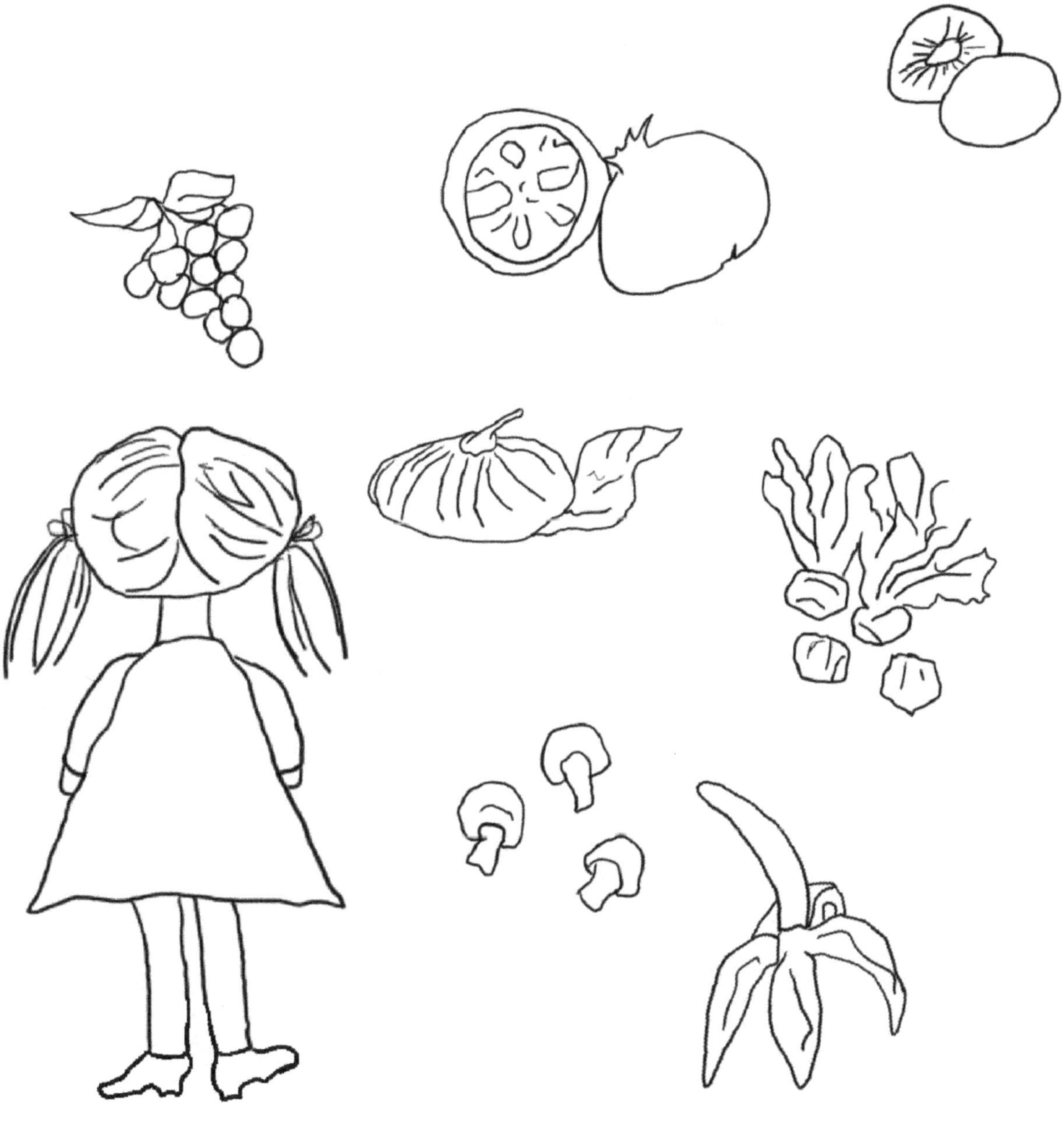

Remember 5 fruits or veggies a day
keeps sickness away!

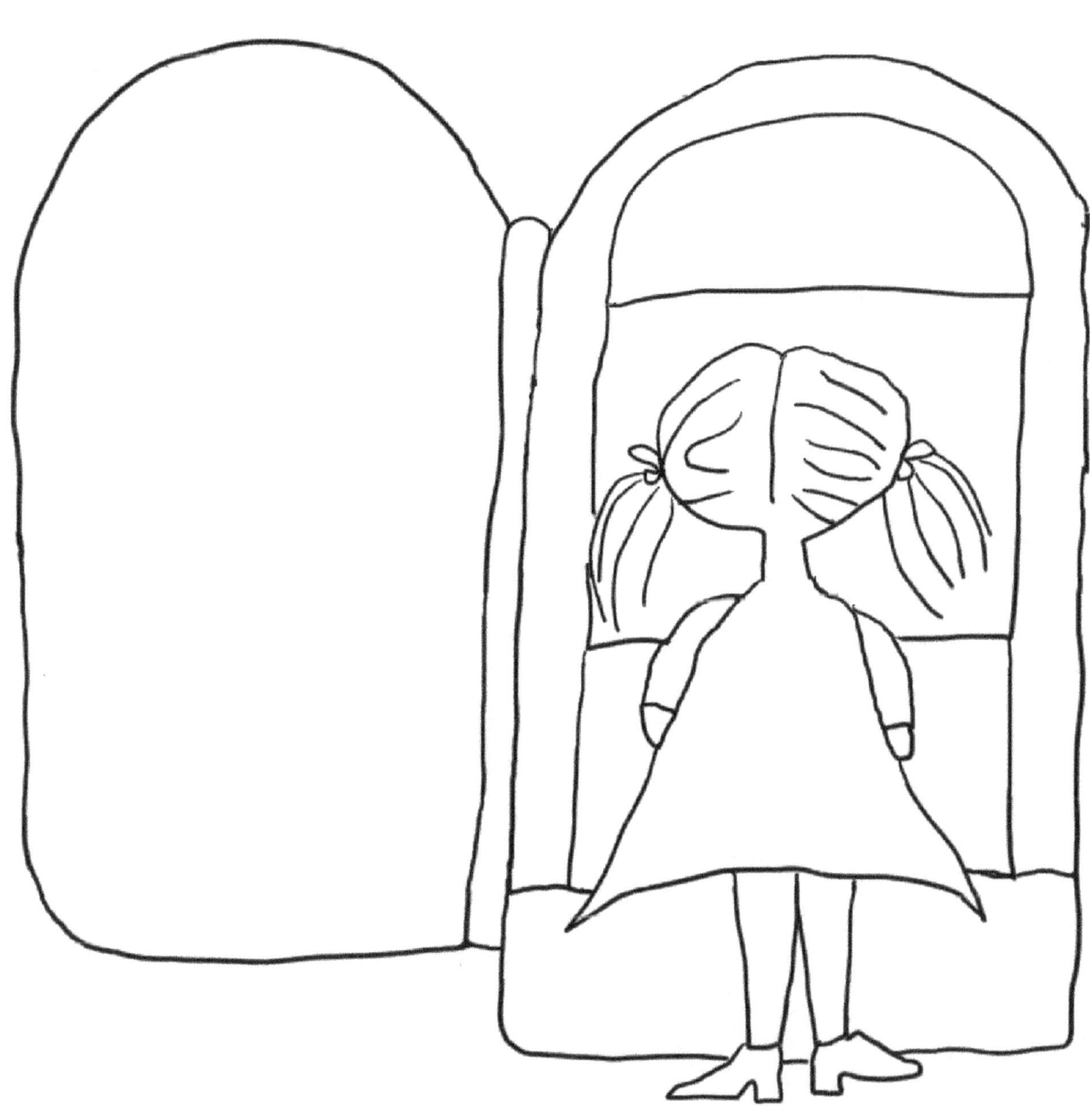

Mom and dad, if you worry about cost,
don't fret. Buy in season or frozen,
for the best value yet.
If you worry about pesticides and
the cost of organic is high,
wash them a minute, and kiss the bad stuff
goodbye!

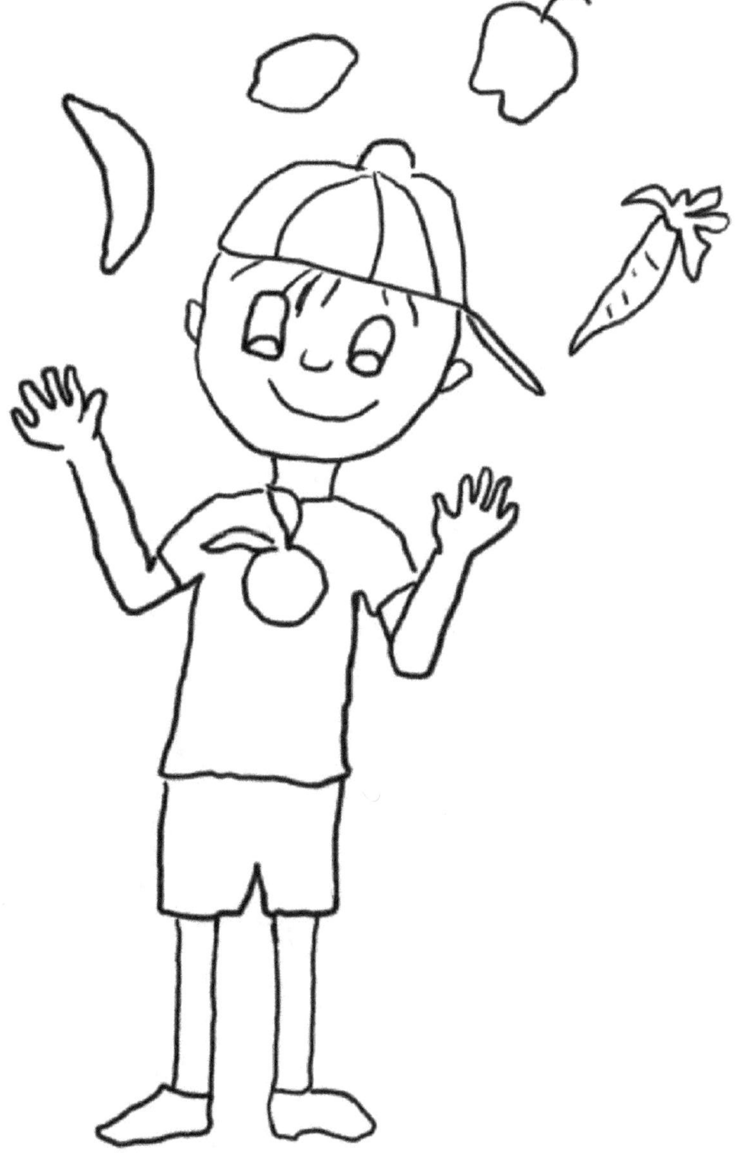